# COMMON SENSE:

# THE CASE FOR AND AGAINST MEDICARE FOR ALL

## LEADING ISSUE
### in the
## 2020 ELECTIONS

by
**John Geyman, M.D.**

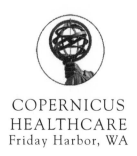

COPERNICUS
HEALTHCARE
Friday Harbor, WA

COMMON SENSE

THE CASE FOR AND AGAINST
MEDICARE FOR ALL:

LEADING ISSUE
in the
2020 ELECTIONS

John Geyman, M.D.

Copernicus Healthcare
Friday Harbor, WA

First Edition
Copyright ©2019 by John Geyman, M.D. All rights reserved

Booklet design, cover and illustrations by W. Bruce Conway
Author photo by Anne Sheridan

softcover: ISBN 78-1-938218-23-1

Library of Congress Control Number is
Available Upon Request From the Publisher

Copernicus Healthcare
34 Oak Hill Drive
Friday Harbor, WA 98250

www.copernicus-healthcare.org

# NOTE TO THE READER

In his famous pamphlet, *Common Sense,* written for the people of the Thirteen Colonies in 1775-1776, Thomas Paine made a strong case to gain independence from England with this opening statement:

> *In the following pages I offer nothing more than **simple facts, plain arguments, and common sense;** and have no other preliminaries to settle with the reader, than to divest himself from prejudice and prepossession, and suffer his reason and his feelings to determine for themselves . . . and generally enlarge his views beyond the present day.*

In this pamphlet, I also offer ***simple facts, plain arguments, and common sense*** about the current crisis in health care in this country and urgent need for reform.

The future of U. S. health care was a leading issue during the 2018 mid-terms, and promises to be even more so as the 2020 election cycle heats up. It becomes more obvious every day that our profit-driven health care marketplace takes health care prices ever upward, therefore more unaffordable and inaccessible for much of our population. Despite temporary short-term improvements under the Affordable Care Act (ACA), major health care reform is again on the table.

Although a bill for single-payer Medicare for All has been in the House of Representatives since 2003 as H.R. 676, initially sponsored by Rep. John Conyers (Dem. MI), it never came to a hearing, was not cleared by committee or brought to the floor for a vote. This year promises to be quite different in

1

the new Democrat-controlled House. The lead sponsor for a new Medicare for All bill in the 116th Congress, Rep. Pramila Jayapal (Dem. WA), has updated the previous H.R. 676 as H.R. 1384. House Speaker Nancy Pelosi has agreed to hold hearings on it in the House. There are now 107 House Democrats in the Medicare for All caucus, while seven in ten Americans support Medicare for All.

As expected, a powerful coalition of corporate stakeholders in the status quo is ready to battle against single-payer as a threat to their medical-industrial complex that profits on the backs of patients, families, and taxpayers. We can expect increasing disinformation from that coalition as well as from many Republicans and the Trump administration.

This pamphlet is targeted to legislators in Congress who will be involved in this new debate over health care, grassroots activists, and the general public seeking to better understand the issues.

The first part describes the new House bill (H.R. 1384). The second part makes the case for single-payer Medicare for All, or national health insurance (NHI), showing how we can well afford to provide universal access to affordable care for all U. S. residents on a long-term sustainable basis while actually saving money. The third part makes the conservative case against single-payer, discrediting myths and disinformation. The fourth part suggests four basic questions that need to be answered in order to effect health care reform.

Note: This pamphlet follows two previous ones, *Common Sense about Health Care Reform in America* (2017) and *More Common Sense: U. S. Health Care at a Crossroads in the 2018 Congress.*

# I. WHAT IS EXPANDED AND IMPROVED MEDICARE FOR ALL?

Expanded and Improved Medicare for All, as described in HR 1384, as soon as it is enacted, will bring:

- A new system of national health insurance (NHI), with equity for all U. S. residents, based on medical need, not ability to pay, and on the principle that health care is not a privilege but a human right.
- Universal access to health care for all U. S. residents, with full choice of providers and hospitals anywhere in the country without any restrictive networks.
- Coverage of all medically necessary care, including outpatient and inpatient services; laboratory and diagnostic services; dental, hearing, and vision care; prescription drugs; reproductive health; maternity and newborn care; mental health services, including substance abuse treatment; and long-term care and supports.
- No cost-sharing such as copays and deductibles at the point of care; no more pre-authorizations or other restrictions now imposed by private insurers.
- Pharmaceutical reform, including negotiated drug prices.
- Administrative simplification with efficiencies and cost containment through large-scale cost controls, including (a) negotiated fee schedules for physicians and other health professionals, who will remain in private practice; (b) global budgeting of individual hospitals and other facilities; and (c) bulk purchasing of drugs and medical devices.

3

- Elimination of the private health insurance industry, with its large administrative overhead and profiteering, and employer-sponsored health insurance.
- Cost savings that enable universal coverage through a not-for-profit single-payer financing system.
- Regional funding for rural and urban areas that are medically underserved.
- Improved quality of care and outcomes for both individuals and populations due to universal access to care.
- Two-year transition period; one year after enactment, U. S. residents over 55 and under 19 will be covered.
- Shared risk for the costs of illness and accidents across the entire population of 326 million.

H. R. 1384 will preserve the separate Veterans Administration and Indian Health Service, and also override the Hyde amendment that bans public funding of abortion.

National polls show that 70 percent of Americans support Medicare for All, including 85 percent of Democrats and a majority of Republicans. [1] A recent Politico/Harvard survey shows that 84 percent of Democrats want Medicare for All to be urgently pursued as an "extremely important priority." [2]

## References
1. Cortez, Z. 2019: The Year for Medicare for All. *Common Dreams*, January 2, 2019.
2. Queally, J. Democrats don't just support Medicare for All, 84% in new poll want party leaders to make it 'extremely important priority.' *Common Dreams*, January 8, 2019.

## II. THE CASE FOR EXPANDED AND IMPROVED MEDICARE FOR ALL

This part has just one goal: to make the case for Medicare for All, or National Health Insurance (NHI).

Here are ten major reasons why we need Medicare for All, as a high priority.

**1. Medicare for All will bring us a system approach to assure access to affordable health care for everyone.**

We cannot contain health care costs that are spiraling out of control without changing our financing system from the current multi-payer system with some 1,300 private insurers to a not-for-profit single-payer system. This will bring a fundamental change in how we finance and pay for health care services.

Recent decades of experience have shown that supposedly competitive markets have wide latitude to set their own prices and that cost containment is nowhere in sight. The private health insurance industry receives $685 billion in government (taxpayer) subsidies each year; the Congressional Budget Office (CBO) projects that this will double over the next ten years. [1] These insurers have segmented the market to their advantage, and without these large subsidies are on a death march still under-recognized by many policymakers and legislators.

**2. The private multi-payer insurance system has failed.**

Medicare for All will be a simplified system, with much less bureaucracy, waste, and fraud. The growth of managed care since the late 1980s and 1990s led to bloated administrative bureaucracies as health maintenance organizations (HMOs) were marketed as new investor-owned companies. An ever-larger administrative bureaucracy was needed to set limits on referrals and hospitalizations, deny services, and dis-enroll sick enrollees. When the insurance market declined by one percent between 2000 and 2005, its workforce grew by one-third! [2]

Since 2010, the ACA has increased bureaucracy further as the exchanges became involved with such activities as determining eligibility for qualified health plans and subsidies/tax credits, as well as verifying annual household income and family size, which are subject to change from year to year. [3]

Over the last two years under the Trump administration, the bureaucracy of health care, especially in the private sector, has become even worse. Privatized Medicaid plans, for example, are experimenting with work requirements in some states. This is a flawed policy from the get-go, since many Medicaid beneficiaries are already working, while many others cannot work due to illness, disability, caring for parents or children, or lack of available jobs in their area. For those who do gain work, ongoing monitoring will be needed since many of their jobs are hourly or temporary and subject to change from one month to another. [4] This adds more bureaucracy.

The administrative overhead of private insurers generally runs between 18 and 20 percent, compared to 2.5 percent for traditional public Medicare. Beyond these high and wasteful administrative costs, private insurers have a long history of profiteering as they feed at the public trough for their government subsidies. As just one of many examples, Tennessee Medicaid plans, operated by Blue Cross Blue Shield of Tennessee, UnitedHealthcare, and Anthem, took in new profits even as they had inadequate physician networks, long waits for care, and denials of many treatments. [5] Private managed care plans frequently game the system for increased revenues by such means as falsifying records, colluding bid-rigging, and withholding payments to providers or subcontractors. Overpayments are common for both privatized Medicare and Medicaid. In more than 30 states, privatized Medicaid plans are endemic, often involving unnecessary or duplicative payments to providers. [6]

**3. Universal coverage through Medicare for All can be paid for by savings, plus moderate progressive taxes.**

Patients, families, and taxpayers can afford Medicare for All. We have had two major studies that tell us for sure that universal coverage through Medicare for All can be largely paid for by savings. The first study by Gerald Friedman, professor of economics at the University of Massachusetts, projected in 2013 that NHI will save about $592 billion annually by cutting out administrative waste of private insurers ($476 billion) and reducing pharmaceutical prices to European levels ($116 billion) through negotiated drug prices and bulk purchasing. [7]

A typical working family of four with employer-sponsored health insurance today pays $28,000 a year for insurance and health care. [8] As a result of the above savings with NHI, 95 percent of Americans would pay less in taxes than they do now for insurance and health care through a progressive tax plan. Those with annual incomes of $50,000 would pay $1,500 in taxes, increasing to $6,000 for incomes of $100,000 and $12,000 for incomes of $200,000 a year. A 2017 update of this study broke down the annual savings of NHI in more detail, as shown in Table 1. [9]

TABLE 1

## Annual Savings With Single-Payer Reform

(In Billions)

| | |
|---|---|
| Insurance overhead & administration of public programs | 220.0 |
| Hospital administration and billing | 149.3 |
| Physicians' office administration and billing | 75.3 |
| Total administration | 503.6 |
| Outpatient prescription drugs | 113.2 |
| Total administration plus outpatient prescription drugs | 616.8 |

Source: Woolhandler, S, Himmelstein, DU. Single-payer reform: The only way to fulfill the President's pledge of more coverage, better benefits, and lower costs. *Annals of Internal Medicine online*, February 21, 2017.

The second study, released on November 30, 2018, by the Political Economy Research Institute (PERI), at the University of Massachusetts-Amherst, finds that single-payer NHI will save the U. S. $5.1 trillion over a decade through savings from multi-payer health care spending in our current profit-driven market-based system. The PERI study estimates that total annual health care spending will increase from $3.2 trillion to $3.6 trillion due to many people getting care that they previously had to forgo. However, that number would be reduced to $2.93 trillion a year by massive savings in administrative, pharmaceutical, and provider payment spending.[10]

Table 2 shows how families will be impacted during the transition to Medicare for All. Lower and middle income families will spend much less for health care under Medicare for All, while high income families will pay only a small amount more.

Present government spending for health care accounts for more than 60 percent of total annual health care costs. The Friedman and PERI studies both rely on new progressive taxes to offset the increased costs of providing universal coverage to all U. S. residents. They would do so by different kinds of taxes, as shown in Table 3.

TABLE 2

# Health Care Spending by Family Income
# Under Medicare for All

| | Health care spending as share of income | | 3. Change in health care spending as share of income (= column 2 − column 1) |
|---|---|---|---|
| | 1. Existing system | 2. Medicare for All | |
| **Low-income families** | | | |
| $13,000 in income with Medicaid | 3.5% | -0.1% | -3.7% |
| $35,000 in income, uninsured | 2.5% | 1.7% | -0.8% |
| **Middle-income families:** $60,000 in income | | | |
| Underinsured | 8.0% | 1.6% | -6.4% |
| Individually insured | 15.5% | 1.6% | -14.0% |
| Insured by employer | 4.2% | 1.6% | -2.6% |
| **High-income families** | | | |
| Top 20 percent: $221,000 in income | -0.1% | 3.7% | +3.9% |
| Top 5 percent: $401,000 in income | -0.9% | 4.7% | +5.6% |

Source: Pollin, R, Heintz, J, Arno, P et al. *In-Depth Analysis by Team of UMass Amherst Economists Shows Viability of Medicare for All.* Amherst, MA, November 30, 2018.

**4. Employers will be relieved of the burden of providing health insurance, will gain a healthier workforce, and be better able to compete in global markets.**

Employers are increasingly frustrated and burdened by the rising costs of providing health insurance for their employees. Under Medicare for All, that burden will be removed as all U. S. residents gain coverage under a new, more efficient system. Most businesses will save money with this change. The auto industry is an example: Ford pays more for its employees' health insurance than it does for the steel to make its cars. The three major auto manufacturers (Ford, GM, and Daimler-Chrysler) have all publicly endorsed Canada's single-payer system from a business and financial standpoint. [11]

## TABLE 3

### Recommended Progressive Taxes By Two Studies Of Medicare For All

| FRIEDMAN STUDY | PERI STUDY |
|---|---|
| 1. Tobin tax of 0.5% on stock trades and 0.01% per year to maturity on transactions in bond, swaps, and trades. | 1. Business premiums set at 8 percent below what a business now spends on health care. |
| 2. 6% surtax on household incomes over $225,000. | 2. 3.75 percent sales tax on nonessential goods. |
| 3. 6% tax on property income from capital gains, dividends, interest, or profits. | 3. Recurring tax of 0.36 percent on all wealth over $1 million. |
| 4. 6% payroll tax on top 60% with incomes over $53,000. | 4. Taxing long-term capital gains as regular income. |
| 5. 3% payroll tax on bottom 40% with incomes under $53,000. | |

**5. Physicians and other health professionals will have more time for patient care, with increased job satisfaction and less burnout.**

Physicians and other health professionals are burdened today with time-consuming billing and clerical tasks that reduce their time for patient care. The cost of billing activities performed by primary care physicians is more than $99,000 a year per physician! [12] A 2017 report from the National Academy of Medicine found that more than one-half of U. S. physicians are exhibiting signs of burnout, including a "high degree of emotional exhaustion and a low sense of personal accomplishment." [13] With simplified Medicare for All, health professionals will have more clinical autonomy, and will no longer have to deal with pre-authorizations and other restrictions imposed by private insurers.

**6. Single-payer NHI will improve the quality of health care for all U. S. residents.**

As soon as Medicare for All is enacted, about 30 million uninsured and perhaps as many as 80 million underinsured will gain access to necessary health care wherever they live, without restrictive networks or out-of-pocket costs at the point of service. Since health insurance is no longer dependent on employment, individuals who lose or change jobs will be covered.

That will make a huge difference, with people no longer delaying or forgoing care, and taking advantage of preventive care and earlier diagnosis and treatment of illness. We could anticipate that the U. S. for the first time will improve its ranking now at the bottom for quality of care compared to ten other advanced countries as measured by regular ongoing cross-national studies by the Commonwealth Fund.

**7. Long-standing gaps in coverage for women's health care, mental health, and rural health care will be corrected.**

The ACA, both before and after GOP sabotage, left gaps in coverage for some essential health care services, exacerbated by policies of the Trump administration. Despite being a majority of the U. S. population, women's health care leads the list of these gaps. Compared to men, women are more likely to have lower wages and incomes, to be on Medicaid (40 million women), and to be the primary caretakers of their children. They are therefore more vulnerable to cuts in safety net and family planning programs than men. [14] Single-payer NHI would improve women's health by mandating all essential reproductive care and remove barriers to all forms of contraception. [15]

Our mental health care system is broken, even for people with health insurance. Many private insurers exclude mental health services. Those plans that do include mental health typically have very restricted numbers of psychiatrists and other mental health providers in their networks. Many psychiatrists and psychologists will not accept new patients, partly because of low reimbursement that doesn't cover their costs. Because of limited access to mental health care, many patients end up in jail as mental health problems become criminalized. [16]

Rural health care has been especially hard hit in recent years. Hospitals are the hub of accessible health care in most large rural areas, where they tend to be the largest employer, but are under-reimbursed. More than 80 have closed since 2010, especially in states that did not expand Medicaid as part of the ACA, with hundreds more rural hospitals at risk for closure. [17] These closures leave a serious shortage of obstetric, trauma and other urgently needed care in their wake. Medicare for All can stabilize these hospitals and help to relieve shortages in health care professionals.

## 8. Disparities across populations based on socio-economic determinants will be reduced.

Disparities have been increasing in our dysfunctional, profit-driven system, thereby resulting in a higher burden of illness, disability, and mortality experienced by one population group compared to another. These disparities are based on socioeconomic determinants, such as income, race/ethnicity, age, gender, disability status, and location. These disparities vary widely from one state to another. As one example, low-income adults in Alabama are almost seven times more likely than high-income people to report skipping needed care because of cost. [18] These disparities will be greatly reduced when all U. S. residents have their Medicare for All card to access care wherever they live.

**9. Oversight of providers and facilities will be improved in terms of patient safety and standards of care.**

As U. S. health care transitions to a single-payer financing system, it will improve the capacity of government to oversee facilities and providers in the public interest. The regulatory process in our present largely privatized, profit-driven system has been far too lax, as well as ineffective. It has been hijacked by corporate stakeholders protecting their revenues in our free-wheeling market-based system. Health care is being treated as just another commodity for sale on an open market. Under NHI, the incentives will change to maximizing efficiency and service for patients, instead of profits to corporate stakeholders.

**10. Single-payer Medicare for All will be sustainable on a long-term basis.**

Instead of the instability and volatility of the current dysfunctional health care "system," besieged as it is with uncontrolled costs as far as the eye can see, NHI will give us a stable system that will control costs on a basis that patients, families, and taxpayers can afford indefinitely into the future. NHI will join Social Security and traditional Medicare as forms of social insurance which depend, by law, for ongoing required contributions by its beneficiaries in order to provide long-term stability.

# References

1. Ockerman, E. It costs $685 billion a year to subsidize U. S. health insurance. *Bloomberg News*, May 23, 2018.
2. Krugman, P. The world of U. S. health care economics is downright scary. *Seattle Post Intelligencer*, September 26, 2006: B1.
3. Office of the Inspector General. Not all of the federally facilitated marketplace's internal controls were effective in ensuring that individuals were properly determined eligible for qualified health plans and insurance affordability programs. Department of Health and Human Services, Washington, D.C., August 2015.
4. Corcoran, M. Medicaid work requirements: Trump's war on the poor expands, one state at a time. *Truthout*, April 25, 2018.
5. Himmelstein, DU, Woolhandler, S. The post-launch problem: the Affordable Care Act's persistently high administrative costs. *Health Affairs Blog*, May 27, 2015.
6. Herman, B. Medicaid's unmanaged managed care. *Modern Healthcare*, April 30, 2016.
7. Friedman, G. Funding H. R. 676: The Expanded and Improved Medicare for All Act. How we can afford a national single-payer health plan. *Physicians for a National Health Program*. July 31, 2013.
8. Girod, GS, Hart, SK, Weldz, SA. 2018 Milliman Medical Index. *Milliman Research Report*, May 21, 2018.
9. Woolhandler, S, Himmelstein, DU. Single-payer reform: The only way to fulfill the President's pledge of more coverage, better benefits, and lower costs. *Annals of Internal Medicine online*, February 21, 2017.
10. Higginbotham, T. Medicare for All is even better than you thought. *Jacobin*, December 3, 2018.
11. Single-payer myths; single-payer facts. Chicago, IL. Physicians for a National Health Program.

12. Tseng, P, Kaplan, RS, Richman, JD et al. Administrative costs associated with physician billing and insurance-related activities at an academic health care system. *JAMA,* February 20, 2018.

13. Clinician well-being is essential for safe, high-quality health care. *National Academy of Medicine.* Washington, D.C., 2017.

14. Bernstein, J, Katch, H. Cutting support for economically vulnerable women is no way to celebrate Mother's Day. *The Washington Post,* May 11, 2018.

15. West, E. Why single-payer is a feminist issue. *Truthout,* January 21, 2018.

16. Gorman, A. Use of psychiatric drugs soars in California jails. *Kaiser Health News,* May 8, 2018.

17. Frakt, A. A sense of alarm as rural hospitals keep closing. *New York Times,* October 29, 2018.

18. 2018 Scorecard on State Health System Performance. New York. *The Commonwealth Fund.*

# III. THE CASE AGAINST MEDICARE FOR ALL: REFUTING MYTHS AND DISINFORMATION

In this part, the case against Medicare for All (NHI) is summarized, including refutation of myths and disinformation perpetuated by its opponents.

## 1. The free market can fix our problems.

Pro-market enthusiasts have argued for decades that a private competitive market exists in health care, and that competition should be allowed to work its wonders. Compared to government or public programs, we are told that the private sector is more efficient and better able to offer value. But it is now obvious over the last 30 to 40 years that competition does not work in health care markets as it does in others. Instead we have increasing consolidation among corporate giants with wide latitude to set prices as they gain market share. Prices are not transparent to the public, whether for outpatient care, hospital services, prescription drugs, or other services, so patients cannot "shop" for care as they do for cars or refrigerators.

Based on experience alone, we can see that free market policies have led to our current, increasing problems of inadequate access, uncontrolled costs, and unacceptable quality of care for our population. Privatized Medicare and Medicaid cost more, are less efficient, and have lower quality of care than their public counterparts.

Joseph Stiglitz, Ph.D., Nobel Laureate in Economics and former chief economist at the World Bank, recognized this disconnect long ago:

*Markets do not lead to efficient outcomes, let alone outcomes that comport with social justice. As a result, there is often good reason for government intervention to improve the efficiency of the market. Just as the Great Depression should have made it evident that the market does not work as well as its advocates claim, our recent Roaring Nineties should have made it self-evident that the pursuit of self-interest does not necessarily lead to overall economic efficiency.* [1]

## 2. Medicare for All is socialism.

This label has a long history in this country, starting with Republican leaders lambasting the New Deal in the 1930s as Bolshevism-lite, continuing into the 1960s with Ronald Reagan warning that Medicare would lead to a socialist dystopia, and now with the GOP and Trump administration calling single-payer NHI a socialist scheme. [2] The National Health Service in England, one of the best health care systems in the world, *is* socialist, with physician practices, hospitals, and other health care facilities government owned and operated. That is also true of our Veterans Administration, which has done such a good job for our veterans over many years. With Medicare for All, however, physicians and other health professionals remain in private practice, with hospitals and other facilities in private hands with global budgets from the government on a year to year basis.

Actually, Medicare for All as NHI is far from a socialist or radical idea. Conservatives in other advanced countries around the world have long supported universal access to necessary

17

health care on the basis of *four conservative moral principles*—anti-free-riding, personal integrity, equal opportunity, and just sharing.

Donald Light, Ph.D., co-author of the important 1996 book, *Benchmarks for Fairness in Health Care Reform,* later laid out these timeless guidelines for conservatives to stay true to their principles:

1. "Everyone is covered, and everyone contributes in proportion to his or her income.
2. Decisions about all matters are open and publicly debated. Accountability for costs, quality, and value of providers, suppliers, and administrators is public.
3. Contributions do not discriminate by type of illness or ability to pay.
4. Coverage does not discriminate by type of illness or ability to pay.
5. Coverage responds first to medical need and suffering.
6. Nonfinancial barriers by class, language, education, and geography are to be minimized.
7. Providers are paid fairly and equitably, taking into account their local circumstances.
8. Clinical waste is minimized through public health, self-care, prevention, strong primary care, and identification of unnecessary procedures.
9. Financial waste is minimized through simplified administrative arrangements and strong bargaining for good value.
10. Choice is maximized in a common playing field where 90-95 percent of payments go to necessary and efficient health services and only 5-10 percent to administration." [3]

## 3. Single-payer NHI will be a government takeover.

Instead of being a government takeover, NHI will be much less bureaucratic compared to today's profit-driven multi-payer system. Health professionals, hospitals, and other providers will have much more time and responsibility for their own day-to-day operations and governance. They will find reimbursement for their services fair, stable, and predictable, a welcome change from the very intrusive dealings with today's private insurers and government requirements at both state and federal levels. NHI, as social insurance against the the financial risk and costs of health care for our entire population, will bring solid protection into the long-term future in the same way that Social Security has since 1935. [4]

## 4. Medicare for All will break the bank.

As described earlier, we have two solid studies of the costs of NHI which find that they can be afforded through *savings* from our present system together with    moderate, progressive taxes that collectively are less than what 95 percent of Americans now pay for insurance and health care.

Some critics claim that patients will abuse the system through overutilization. Indeed, we can expect some increased utilization when so many millions of uninsured and underinsured Americans gain access to essential care that they had delayed or avoided due to costs. The PERI study already factored in an increase of about 12 percent in utilization after NHI is launched while acknowledging that this is probably a "high end" estimate. As the researchers stated in their extensive 198-page 2018 report:

*Experience in Canada, as well as in the U. S. with the implementation of Medicare, suggests that the finite supply of hospital beds and physician time dampens increases in the society-wide use of care. Indeed, in those past cases, the increases in utilization by previously uninsured groups were offset by small decreases in utilization among those who had been covered prior to the reforms, resulting in no overall increase in the number of hospitalizations or physician visits.*[5]

## 5. Wait times will be too long.

This is not a credible claim since there are so many people today, both with and without insurance, who face long wait times, often without *ever* getting an appointment! Even if a patient gets an appointment, wait times can be very lengthy. Four years after the ACA was passed, a 2014 report found that the national average wait time to see a cardiologist in Washington, D.C. was 32 days and 66 days to schedule a physician examination in Boston (despite being the city with the most physicians per capita, mostly non-primary care specialists). [6] About one-third of U. S. physicians won't see a new patient on Medicaid. Yes, patients can be seen in an E.R., but follow-up appointments with practicing physicians typically are very difficult and time-consuming to arrange.

It is true that patients can wait for long periods in Canada to see specialists for *elective* procedures, but patients with emergency or urgent conditions will be seen immediately there and in other single-payer countries.

## 6. Medicare for All (NHI) will bring rationing.

This is a common myth perpetuated by opponents of NHI. It is completely the opposite—NHI will assure access to all necessary care for all U. S. residents, regardless of age, pre-existing conditions, or location in the country. Meanwhile, this myth has become a meme, fueled by corporate stakeholders in the present profit-driven market-based system, who deny that rationing occurs every day. Here are just some of the ways that care is rationed now:

- All the millions of uninsured and underinsured who can't afford care.
- Denial of services by insurers.
- Insurers placing cancer and other specialized drugs in top tiers that are unaffordable even for the insured.
- Disenrollment of sicker patients in privatized Medicare and Medicaid programs.
- Restrictive coverage by insurers for women's health care and mental health services.

## 7. Enacting Medicare for All will be too disruptive.

Conservatives, who want to keep the status quo with all its problems, argue that such a fundamental change as single-payer financing of health care will be much too disruptive. Others, including many Democrats, promote incremental change, such as rebuilding the ACA, which largely failed to reform our system and can never bring universal coverage.

In response, how can U. S. health care be more disruptive than it is now?! Instead, single-payer NHI will immediately start to correct today's system problems, in the same seamless way that Medicare and Medicaid did when they were enacted in the mid-1960s. Then, patients went to physicians and hospitals with their new cards and were accepted for care without questions. Today, everyone will have a Medicare for All card as our current financial barriers to care go away.

Admittedly, there will be plenty of disruption in the bloated private administrative sector, but that is needed to rectify its many problems that have been sold to us under the false banner of "more efficiency in the private sector."

**8. What will happen to all the displaced workers in the private insurance industry?**

Yes, the 1.7 million workers displaced by single-payer will have to look for new jobs, but many can be retrained in the expanded public sector implementing NHI. That, however, is a much lower number than the 60 million Americans who are separated from their jobs each year. H.R. 1384 allocates 1 percent of its budget over the first five years for assistance and retraining of workers displaced by elimination of the private health insurance industry.

In summary, Medicare for All will be an essential advance for all U. S. residents and the nation. There will be winners and losers, as Table 4 shows, but this will be as important an advance as Social Security was in 1935.

Table 4

# Winners and Losers under Single-Payer Medicare for All

| Winners | Losers |
|---|---|
| All Americans | Private health insurers |
| Physicians, other health professionals | Corporate middlemen |
| Hospitals | Corporate stakeholders |
| Employers | Privatized Medicare |
| Mental health care | Privatized Medicaid |
| Public health | Displaced workers |
| Federal and state governments | Lobbyists |
| Taxpayers | |

Source: Geyman, JP. *TrumpCare: Lies, Broken Promises, How It Is Failing and What Should Be Done. Copernicus Healthcare*, Friday Harbor, WA, 2018, p.246.

## *Conclusion:*

Other competing proposals to health care reform are being brought forward in the 116th Congress, such as ways to repair some of the damage the GOP has wrought to the Affordable Care Act (ACA). Others may use variants of the name Medicare for All, such as "Medicare Extra for All," Medicare buy-in at age 55, or other variations that do not assure universal coverage. [7]

None of those incremental proposals, however, can effectively address the nation's serious problems of inadequate access to affordable health care. Fundamental financing reform, as represented by real Medicare for All (NHI), is the *only* way that we can achieve universal coverage that is accessible and affordable for all of us.

# References:

1. Stiglitz, JE. Evaluating economic change. *Daedlalus* 133/3, Summer 2004.
2. O'Brien, M. Giving everyone health care doesn't make you a communist. *The Washington Post*, October 25, 2018.
3. Light, DW. A conservative call for universal access to health care. *Penn Bioethics* 9 (4): 4-6, 2002.
4. Marmor, TR. Social insurance and American health care: Principles and paradoxes. *Journal of Health Politics, Policy and Law*. December 2018.
5. Pollin, R, Heintz, J, Arno, P et al. *In-Depth Analysis by Team of UMass Amherst Economists Shows Viability of Medicare for All*. Amherst, MA, November 30, 2018.
6. Rosenthal, E. The health care waiting game. *New York Times*, July 5, 2014.
7. Kishore, S, Johnson, M, Berwick, D. What do the midterms mean for Medicare for All? *Health Affairs Blog*, December 3, 2018.

## IV. HOW SHOULD WE DECIDE?

If you as an individual or in an organization had the opportunity to recommend and/or the authority to determine who should have health insurance, how would you decide? And further, how would you decide who should *not* have health insurance? If you were meeting face to face with the people in the U. S., who would you tell they *cannot* have health insurance

We all should become well versed in the substance of the current H. R. 1384, Expanded and Improved Medicare for All, as put forward by its lead sponsor, Rep. Pramila Jayapal (Dem. WA). The press will be following its hearings in the House, its progress through committees, and hopefully to a vote in the Democrat-controlled floor of the House of Representatives. Health care will be a leading issue across the country as campaigns proceed at state and national levels in the 2020 election cycle. As we study the arguments for and against Medicare for All, the resources listed in Part V will be useful.

We should all be asking these four basic questions which need answers:

1. *Who is the health care system for?* Is it for patients and families or corporate stakeholders in the medical-industrial complex?
2. *Should health care services be not-for-profit—or for-profit as just another commodity on an open market?*
3. *Is health care a human right or a privilege based on ability to pay?*
4. *What ethic should prevail in health care: a business "ethic" maximizing revenue to providers or a service ethic based on needs of patients and families?*

Most advanced countries around the world answered these questions many years ago. The U. S. remains an outlier among other advanced countries in still not assuring universal access to health care. Western Europe and Scandinavian countries all have systems of universal health care, as do Canada, New Zealand, Australia, Taiwan, and other countries. Health care was recognized as a human right way back in 1948, when the General Assembly of the United Nations adopted its Universal Declaration of Human Rights, which was also later adopted by the World Health Organization in its Declaration of the Rights of Patients.

We can, and should, learn from the wisdom of leaders in past years. Dr. Henry Sigerist, Director of the History of Medicine at the Johns Hopkins University, made this key observation as far back as 1944, still very relevant today:

> *Illness is an unpredictable risk for the individual family, but we know fairly accurately how much illness a large group of people will have, how much medical care they will require, and how many days they will have to spend in hospitals. In other words, we cannot budget the cost of illness for the individual family but we can budget it for the nation. The principle must be to spread the risk among as many people as possible . . . The experience of the last 15 years in the United States has, in my opinion, demonstrated that voluntary health insurance does not solve the problem of the nation. It reaches only certain groups and is always at the mercy of economic fluctuations . . . Hence, if we decide to finance medical services through insurance, the insurance system must be compulsory.*[1]

We need to build on grassroots activism and broad public support for NHI. To be sure, powerful corporate interests across the medical-industrial complex, together with their Wall Street allies, are assembling their wagons once again to defeat real health care reform. They will fight hard to maintain their very profitable control over U. S. health care, and will have unlimited money to fund their campaign. We can expect all kinds of disinformation and lies about Medicare for All.

As the debate goes forward, we should not give credence to sound-alike proposals that introduce facsimile alternatives to Medicare for All (NHI). The Democrats themselves may be their own worst enemy in this respect. Already some leading Democrats in Congress are voicing support of some of these alternatives, such as expanding the public option, introducing new buy-ins to Medicare, expansion of Medicare Advantage, and letting employers offer their own private health plans. (2) However, none of these alternatives will bring universal coverage, the profiteering private insurance industry remains in place, containment of health care costs will be inadequate, complex bureaucracy will continue, and many millions of Americans will be uninsured or underinsured.

A recent report from Gallup News documents that 70 percent of Americans have, over more than 20 years, described the U. S. health care system as being "in a state of crisis" or having "major problems," as shown in Figure 1. [3]

Figure 1

# Ratings of the U. S. Healthcare System, 1994-2018

Which of these statements do you think best describes the U. S. health care system today? It is in a state of crisis/major problems, or it has minor or no problems.

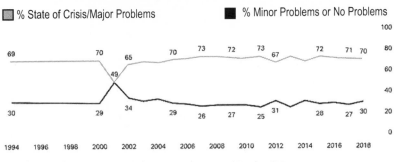

Note: The figure for 2009 is an average of two polls conducted in September and November of that year

Source: Gallup News

We will need an unbiased, objective media to present the real issues to the public, including transparency of deceptive corporate stakeholder lobbying efforts.

The crisis in U. S. health care has become so serious and hurtful to much of our population that we need to make a decision for real reform an urgent priority. As Robert Reich, professor of public policy at the University of California Berkeley, chairman of Common Cause, and author of the new book, *The Common Good*, tells us:

> *The real choice in the future is either a hugely expensive for-profit oligopoly with the market power to charge high prices even to healthy people and stop insuring sick people. Or else a government-run single-payer system—such as is in place in almost every other advanced economy—dedicated to lower premiums and better care for everyone. We're going to have to choose eventually.* [4]

Can the common good prevail through this highly contested political process? Whether or not we can adopt real health care reform through Medicare for All will test our democracy to the core.

### References:

1.  Sigerist, HE. Medical care for all the people. *Canadian Journal of Public Health* 35 (7): 258, 1944.
2.  Rogers, A, Raju, M, Landers, E. Democrats distance themselves from Harris' call to eliminate private health plans. *CNN*, January 30, 2019.
3.  *Gallup News,* as referenced by Conley, J. New analysis shows why Democrats are wrong to fear bold embrace of Medicare for All. *Common Dreams*, January 14, 2019.
4.  Reich, R. Why a single-payer healthcare system is inevitable. *Common Dreams*, August 22, 2016.

# V. USEFUL RESOURCES

## Websites
1. Quote of the Day. don@mccanne.org
2. Physicians for a National Health Program. Chicago, IL. www.pnhp.org
3. HealthCare-NOW. www.healthcare-now.org
4. Copernicus Healthcare. www.copernicus-healthcare.org

## Reports
1. Friedman, G. Funding H. R. 676: The Expanded and Improved Medicare for All Act. How we can afford a national single-payer health plan. Physicians for a National Health Program. July 31, 2013.
2. Pollin, R, Heintz, J, Arno, P et al. *In-Depth Analysis by Team of UMass Amherst Economists Shows Viability of Medicare for All*. Amherst, MA, November 30, 2018.
3. Overall Health System Performance in Eleven Countries. Periodic reports from *The Commonwealth Fund*, New York City, NY.

## Books
1. Geyman, JP. *TrumpCare: Lies, Broken Promises, How It Is Failing and What Should Be Done*. Friday Harbor, WA. *Copernicus Healthcare*, 2018.
2. Geyman, JP. *Crisis in U. S. Health Care: Corporate Power vs. the Common Good*. Friday Harbor, WA. *Copernicus Healthcare*, 2017.
3. Young, Q. *Everybody In Nobody Out: Memoirs of a Rebel Without a Pause*. Friday Harbor, WA. *Copernicus Healthcare*, 2013.

## Articles:
1. Woolhandler, S, Himmelstein, DU. Single-payer reform: The only way to fulfill the President's pledge of more coverage, better benefits, and lower costs. *Annals of Internal Medicine online*, February 21, 2017.
2. Marmor, TR. Social insurance and American health care: Principles and paradoxes. *Journal of Health Politics, Policy and Law.* December 2018.
3. Higginbotham, T. Medicare for All is even better than you thought. *Jacobin*, December 3, 2018

# ABOUT THE AUTHOR

John Geyman, M.D. is professor emeritus of family medicine at the University of Washington School of Medicine in Seattle, where he served as Chairman of the Department of Family Medicine from 1976 to 1990. As a family physician with over 21 years in academic medicine, he also practiced in rural communities for 13 years. He was the founding editor of *The Journal of Family Practice* (1973 to 1990) and the editor of *The* 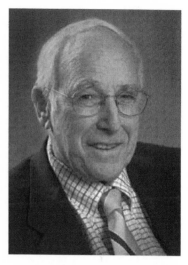 *Journal of the American Board of Family Medicine* from 1990 to 2003. Since 1990 he has been involved with research and writing on health policy and health care reform. He served as president of Physicians for a National Health Program from 2005 to 2007, and is a member of the National Academy of Medicine.

## His books include:

*Struggling and Dying Under TrumpCare: How We Can Fix this Fiasco* (2019)

*Trumpcare: Lies, Broken Promises, How it is Failing, and What Can Be Done* (2018)

*Common Sense: U. S. Health Care at a Crossroads in the 2018 Congress* (Pamphlet, 2018)

*Common Sense about Health Care Reform in America* (Pamphlet, 2017)

*Crisis in U.S Health Care: Corporate Power vs. the Common Good* (2017)

*The Human Face of ObamaCare: Promises vs. Reality and What Comes* Next (2016)

*How ObamaCare is Unsustainable: Why We Need a Single-Payer Solution for All Americans* (2015)

*Souls on a Walk: An Enduring Love Story Unbroken by Alzheimer's* (2012)

*Health Care Wars: How Market Ideology and Corporate Power Are Killing Americans* (2012)

*Breaking Point: How the Primary Care Crisis Endangers the Lives of Americans.* (2011)

*Hijacked: The Road to Single-Payer in the Aftermath of Stolen Health Care Reform* (2010)

*The Cancer Generation: Baby Boomers Facing a Perfect Storm* (2009)

*Do Not Resuscitate: Why the Health Insurance Industry is Dying, and How We Must Replace It* (2008)

*The Corrosion of Medicine: Can the Profession Reclaim Its Moral Legacy?* (2008)

*Shredding the Social Contract: The Privatization of Medicare* (2006)

*Falling Through the Safety Net: Americans Without Health Insurance* (2005)

*The Corporate Transformation of Health Care: Can the Public Interest Still Be Served?* (2004)

*Health Care in America: Can Our Ailing System Be Healed?* (2002)

*Family Practice: Foundation of Changing Health Care* (1985)

*The Modern Family Doctor and Changing Medical Practice* (1971)

Copies of this pamphlet can be ordered from Amazon.com for $5.95, or as a Kindle eBook version at $2.99.

For more background and analysis, copies of my new 2019 book, *Struggling and Dying Under TrumpCare: How We Can Fix This Fiasco*, can also be ordered from Amazon. com ($18.95) or as a Kindle eBook ($2.99).

43376610R00024

Made in the USA
Middletown, DE
24 April 2019